Yoga For Men

A Beginners Guide To Develop Core Strength, Flexibility and Aid Recovery

Jake Bailey

Copyright © HRD Publishing 2015

All rights reserved.

ISBN-13: 978-1517410964
ISBN-10: 1517410967

CONTENTS

1	Introduction	6
2	Why Should Men Do Yoga?	8
3	Yoga Breathing	15
4	Yoga For Focus	18
5	Yoga Exercises	20
6	Deep Relaxation and Recovery	35
7	Summary	39
8	Yoga Resources For Beginners	40

YOGA FOR MEN

INTRODUCTION

Going to your first yoga class might be a little weird, but what isn't weird the first time you try it? Your first day at a new job was little weird because it was new-you didn't know where things were, you didn't know peoples' names and so on. There was a lot to remember and learn, but you survived, you got connected and got comfortable.

Developing a yoga practice isn't really painful, although your poses and routines will be grueling at times. You do have to consider some different things, such as what style of yoga you want to try, which classes you'd like to attend and what poses will compliment you existing athletic regimen.

If there's a new sport you're getting into when you roll out your mat for the first time that can complicate things a bit more. The good news is that yoga is the ideal complement to any athletic activity. This book will give you the guidance you need to understand yoga and develop a sound practice that will yield many benefits for the rest of your life.

What are you going to learn?

I will help you create a yoga practice that will meet your unique needs. Your yoga mat will become your laboratory of transformation. I'll show you how to connect to every muscle in your body and to develop connections between every muscle and muscle group in the same workout. You will learn how to prevent injuries and incorporate your yoga practice into any athletic regimen you are involved in. I'll teach you how to be your own teacher as your yoga practice continues to progress and become an integral part of your life.

This book has been created to help men who've had little or no experience with yoga reach their full potential through simple, effective means.

Are you ready to take on one of the most unique challenges of your life?

Yoga isn't like any other kind of exercise, except that it is just as challenging as anything as any other exercise. With yoga, you will learn how to exercise your mind with your body.

WHY SHOULD MEN DO YOGA?

There's more than one correct answer to this question. Before we start answering them, forget the idea that yoga is a "chick thing" or is only beneficial to women. I don't care how many classes you've seen full of women, you belong on a yoga mat just the same. Forget the idea that yoga is wimpy; one class will cure you of that.

Let's memorize one simple truth as we get started: Real men do Yoga

What is a real man? You are. There's no one definition of a real man. But we all know that any man who has had a real, positive influence in our lives, either when we were boys or when we were fully grown, was one who was disciplined and strong in one way or another. They may not have been star athletes, CEOs or high-ranking public officials, but they were strong in *some way*. We look at such men with respect because we can see they were devoted in some way and manifested their devotion in a meaningful way.

Yoga's influence on today's man

It's been 12 years since John Capouya released a book called Real Men Do Yoga that profiled male athletes who did Yoga. Back then, yoga's popularity was exploding, but athletes weren't really in the media's sights. Time Magazine did a cover story that dwelt in female Hollywood celebrities-supermodel Christy Turlington posed on the cover in Rooster Pose-it was impressive but it was also a pose that only looked impressive if the person doing it was tall and skinny. The article went on to discuss Madonna's spiritual revelations that she got from her new-found yoga practice.

As a result of the media being so focused on women whenever it came to yoga, the male world stayed disconnected from yoga. I can recall telling a male friend over beer after golf one day that I had started doing yoga. He replied by saying that his mother-in-law swore by her yoga, but it would never be 'a guy thing'. A book released in 2003 by John Capouya called Real Men Do Yoga barely raised eyebrows-men just weren't paying attention-except male pro athletes.

Turn the clock back to the late 1980s. American basketball was grabbing attention from all over the world. One of the NBA's greatest stars, both of his time and in hoop history, Kareem Abdul Jabbar, was an avid yoga practitioner. Today, he still practices daily and is, by any standards, in exceptionally good shape-the same way we want to be described when we get older.

"For me I noticed improvement in my posture – that was key for me because I had been having lower back problems," Abdul-Jabbar states. "After I started doing yoga positions – asanas — all that changed. My health greatly improved overall," Abdul-Jabbar told USA Today in 2003.

Abdul-Jabbar's interview by USA Today happened a decade after he retired. They were focusing on how the retired hoop star stayed in such good shape so long after being out of basketball. He played 20 seasons with the NBA.

"I believe that yoga is one of the reasons I was able to play as long and as healthy as I did."

-Kareem Abdul-Jabbar, NBA superstar

Fast forward to 2013. Abdul-Jabbar had long-since been out of basketball, but was and still is into yoga. His son, Amir, is a yoga teacher by trade. Yoga has long since ceased to be a novelty among pro athletes-now it's a mainstream thing.

LeBron James credits yoga with helping him get back on track in last year's NBA championship series.

Ryan Giggs believes yoga was pivotal in extending his soccer career at Manchester United into his 40's. Yoga is now practiced by players of every pro sport.

What are the benefits of yoga in plain English?

Everyone who practices yoga, from the average folks at the gyms we work out in to superstar athletes like Ray Lewis and Evan Longoria, cite the same benefits that yoga gives them.

- Yoga helps you reduce your stress level.
- It teaches you to focus better and more thoroughly.
- You develop better breathing patterns which increase your stamina.
- Better balance and body control come to you through yoga practice.
- You learn how to relax.
- You prevent injuries by restoring mobility and getting to know your body.

You may think you know your body, but once you start doing yoga, you will get to know yourself better than you ever thought you could.

You don't need to be flexible to do yoga

One of the most-common misconceptions among people who've never done yoga is that they think they can't be "good at yoga" because they weren't born flexible. Let's face it-most athletes aren't very flexible, their muscles are tight from repetitive motions of the games they play or the sports they practice.

All athletes who do yoga benefit from yoga. Stretching is just one part of it. The deeper part of practicing yoga is getting your mind to talk to your body and getting your mind to listen to your body when it needs to talk back. When you get on your mat, your mind and body bond and become connected. Your body ceases to be a slave of your mind-you are essentially "clearing your body" the same way you would do some grueling exercise to "clear your head".

Yoga for Balance and Body Control

Every man's yoga practice will be a bit different for the same reason that no two humans are exactly alike, however, every man's yoga practice will include and share certain basic poses and sequences of poses. It is far easier to master some specific poses first and work on breathing techniques later. Why?

Moving our bodies into yoga poses requires us to think about how we're moving and how we are positioned. You don't need to do complicated poses, either, at least not right away. As you develop technique and build confidence in our simple poses, you'll be naturally driven by that confidence to try your technical abilities in more-complex poses. That happens naturally as it does with any discipline you learn.

Warrior II Pose

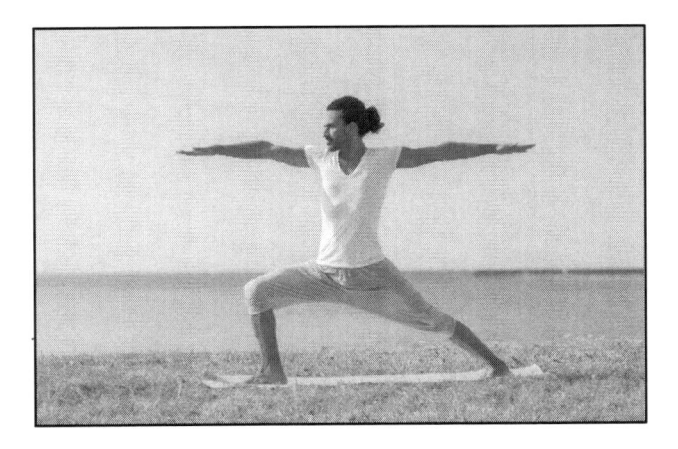

Take a simple pose like warrior II. The first time you do it, you'll notice your thighs burn a bit as the muscles start to work. You have to consciously extend the length of your legs to keep your feet planted. You grab the mat with your toes to engage your ankles and create strength in your stance so that you can drop your weight deeper into the pelvic floor.

The biggest difference between yoga and traditional exercise is that many muscles work at their full, extended length. You work more of the surface area and deep tissue of each muscle. In the end, you work the whole muscle instead of just one part.

As you work the full length of each muscle that's involved with the pose you are doing, you develop a much deeper connection with your body. You become aware of the different muscles, not just because they might be working harder, but because you have to think your way into the pose, and you have to maintain the connections you've just made in order to hold yourself into the position.

Making the mind-body connection in a pose triggers an instinctive, conscious connection with your breathing. Yoga moves fast enough to make you exert energy, but it moves slow enough that you can think about every stage of movement. It is through physical poses that you begin to develop yogic breathing techniques.

Warrior I Pose

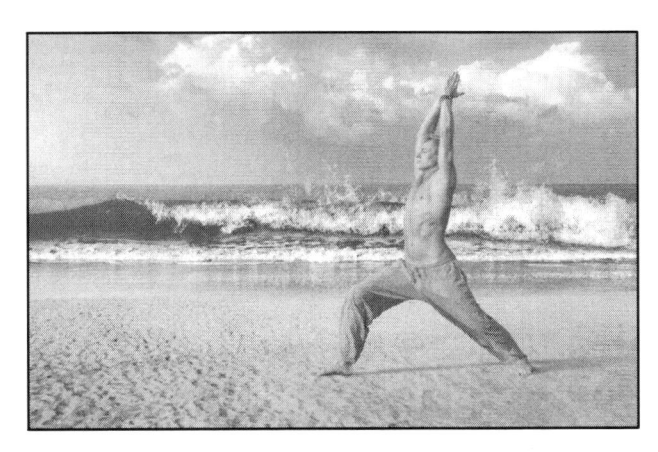

Warrior I pose is very similar to Warrior II. You'll focus on keeping your feet planted, extending your thighs inside and out, and keeping your abdominals gently pulled in so that they support your back and torso. Give it a quick try.

- Stand facing the long side of your mat. Open the feet three to four feet apart.

- Rotate right foot to point forward. Rotate left toes inward.

- Bend right knee and bring directly over ankle. Spin torso to face forward.

- Relax shoulders and raise arms overhead, palms together, gazing up toward hands with relaxed neck.

- Maintain focus on your breathing as you regulate your abs to keep them gently pulled in.

- Repeat on other side.

Your thighs and your buttocks create a pelvic floor of support that holds the weight of your torso. The thigh muscles are extended and engaged in this pose as are the abdominals.

How long should I hold each pose?

There is no one correct answer for this. It will depend on your physical condition, the posture you're doing, and your goals. As a general guide for standing poses, 5 long, slow breaths is a good benchmark to aim for. If you find this too tasking, start at 2 or 3 and work your way up over time. If you're comfortable, take it up to 10 breaths. Listen to your body and respond accordingly.

YOGA BREATHING

Breath control is hard work. Don't let anyone tell you differently. Think back to when you were a child and you were under stress of one kind or another. Someone probably told you: "now, take deep breath". Anxiety isn't something that men usually talk about, but it is something we all feel. When you get stressed out, your breathing gets shallow. You feel like you would if you were laying down and a gorilla was sitting on your chest. No matter how hard you try to breath, your chest still feels tight and you can't seem to take in a good breath of air.

Most of us can't just take control of the pace of our breath, we need to learn some technique to be able to make it happen. The easiest way to start building breath control technique is by doing yoga poses that involve the engagement of the abdominal muscles. That's why the warrior pose is such a good one to start with.

As you get into Warrior and other basic poses for balance and body control, you're going to find it fairly easy to start controlling your breath simply by engaging the abs to hold your body steady. As you pull in your abs to steady your torso, they help lift the diaphragm to push air out of your lungs as you exhale. Ease up on the abdominal pull-in and you help pull the diaphragm drop down to pull air into the lungs as you inhale.

Once you've done the basic poses a few times, you will start to develop the ability to consciously move your abs inward and outward. You'll soon find you can consciously drive the pace of your breath by doing this.

What makes breath control difficult? The science and the yoga of breathing

Breathing is an involuntary function of the body. It is driven by the medulla, the automatic part of the brain that drives the heartbeat. Both breath and heartbeat are influenced by chemicals and hormones produced by the brain, much of which comes from the subconscious mind after the conscious mind observes and processes life experiences at they come at you.

By connecting your automatic breath to our willing, conscious motion- your movement in and out of a yoga pose, you connect your conscious mind to your subconscious mind and your mind and body are then bonded to work together much more closely.

Breath syncing: Try a yoga breathing exercise

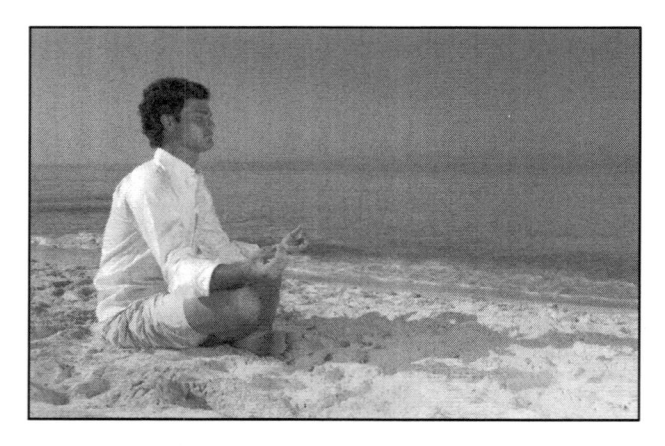

An easy way to learn the concept of yoga breathing is to do simple movements *while* breathing. Sit in *sukhasana* (picture above) and extend your arms out, push all the breath out of your lungs as you gradually bring your arms down outstretched and your hands down to the floor. Then inhale slowly while you move your arms upward so that your palms eventually come together over your head, arms fully stretched.

The idea is to move *with* the pace of your breath, and breathe *with* the pace of your movement. You fill your lungs gradually as your arms are lifting, you sync your arms and your breath so that your lungs are full by the time your palms meet. You subsequently empty your lungs gradually while your arms open up and your hands descend back down. Your lungs should be empty and exhale complete by the time your hands get back down to the floor. The idea is that you breathe consciously, to connect the mind and body.

You can do this kind of synchronized breathing/moving with any motion you like. Pick whichever movement allows the process to be easy. There are no points for overexerting your mind to get the process down. The process is involving enough that you don't have to worry about it being too easy to count as a challenge. Besides, this is a basic concept that will properly *prepare* you for the challenging poses you know you want to do.

Once you start to master breathing in sync with moving, you can start to apply the concept with poses that you will hold, such as the warrior pose we tried before, and many others. In a pose such as warrior, there isn't a wide range of movement once you are in the pose. However, there is really no such thing as standing still in any pose.

Once you are in a pose like warrior, you have to connect with the muscles that are holding you into the position. You want those muscles to stretch out gradually so that you can use the full length of the muscle and not just one small area. You silently talk yourself deeper into the movement. You tell the muscles to stretch a little more, and then hold the position and stretch a bit more. Each time you tell a muscle to stretch and hold, you go through a full breath cycle.

Once you are fully stretched in a pose, you may talk your way through adjustments of your position to make yourself feel more relaxed and comfortable in the pose. You do a breathe cycle each time you do this as well. Throughout this process, you learn to lengthen or shorten your breaths accordingly to increase your level of comfort and deepen the connection between mind and body.

YOGA FOR FOCUS

Yoga for focus is a science that really never stops expanding. The longer you practice yoga, the greater your ability to focus will be. The first aspect of using yoga to develop your ability to focus involves what you just read about breathing. Your conscious connection to your breath, which is an automatic function until you make your connection. This is the first stage in developing the conscious ability to focus. The ability continues to develop as you take your breath control into deep poses-this makes your brain workout with your body, and is an example of the common term "mind-body" exercise.

Think of a place that you go to where you are able to focus better. Maybe it is a quiet room, maybe it is a noisy café where distractions get drowned by the background activity. The point is, there is some place where you find yourself having an easier time focusing on whatever you are doing.

One of the biggest benefits of yoga is that it teaches you to focus from within yourself-it enables you to be less dependent on places or circumstances to get yourself focused. You learn breath control to sync your mind and body, and then you exercise the concept in your poses, so you learn to focus yourself from within yourself, regardless of where you are.

Challenging yoga poses help you further develop your ability to focus. A balancing pose, such as Tree pose or Vrksasana (picture in next Chapter), is an obvious choice because it is a balancing pose. You learn to tweak your muscles to help yourself stay standing. Tree pose also introduces the concept of connecting to the environment around you to increase your focus further. Most people choose something in front of them to look at in order to help engage and focus in the pose. In yoga, the visual focal point is called *dristi*.

When you get into poses that are more grueling or which involve more-complex movement, you start to "learn by doing"-you develop focal ability simply by doing the pose. If you hold a simple pose such as warrior for a long period of time, it becomes grueling. You can make subtle adjustments within the pose to distribute your weight so that muscles don't burn so much.

As you learn this search-and-apply process of finding different muscles and muscle positions, you widen your focal ability. You learn to stay calm in the pose as you look for ways to increase comfort and to strengthen your stance or other position if it is another pose. At this point, your yoga practice becomes like any other task in that you improve your ability through practice and repetition.

The greatest athletes never really stop doing fundamental drills that were part of their practice as beginners. They simply incorporate more knowledge into those drills as they become experienced in their sports. Of course, yoga can stay mellow and be just as effective for you; it doesn't have to be like boot camp if you don't want it to be. If you go to a class where a teacher acts too much like a drill instructor, then find another teacher. If you like the teacher and the class, stay put. Practice at home with the poses and sequences in this book, and you'll get to be your own teacher and mix it up however you want.

YOGA EXERCISES

Yoga exercises continue to gain popularity in the fitness world. One of the best things about yoga is that it will complement any athletic discipline or any other workout routine. If you lift weights or do any other kind strength training, yoga will benefit you by restoring the length of your muscles after a workout.

As you flex and move muscles in strength training, they become shorter and tighter. This puts strain and tendons and, in very extreme cases, can cause the breaking of bones. Also, if muscles are never stretched back to normal length, they too can get injured through strains, tears, and pulls.

Yoga exercises can be easily sequenced so that you can counteract the shortening of muscles right away, in the present tense, by doing a pose that counters the previous pose that you just did before. For example, a pose that bends you back can be countered with a forward bend.

Yoga exercise differs from regular exercise because you engage the muscles more consciously and more slowly so that you literally think through the process of each exercise. In yoga, your body is not a slave to your mind; nor is your mind a slave to your body. Instead, the body is partnered with the mind and they work together to develop the body and a mental connection at the same time.

Each yoga pose will affect you a bit differently. It is important to remember that yoga isn't like other kinds of exercise. This is true not only because the mind is more closely involved with the whole exercise process, but also because the whole body is always involved. Even if the pose is focused primarily on your legs, for example, your arms and neck will still be involved in the pose.

We looked at a couple of poses earlier in our reading; let's look at those poses again and start to tie them into sequences of yoga poses. Basic poses that you learn first will always be the foundation of any yoga practice, no matter how advanced your practice becomes. Your practice will indeed become more advanced in due course.

Yoga is an activity that every person can master. We might not all become exercise gurus, but yoga poses are based on mind-body "programming". Yoga is sort of like a video game in certain aspects. Think about someone you know who is good at a particular video game. Maybe that person is a friend, or maybe that person is you. When a person is good at a video game, you never really describe that person as having "talent" because he can win the game most of the time. He is good at the game because he plays all the time. This is not to say that the game that is mastered isn't challenging. Yoga will challenge you and so will any complex video game. But like a video game, yoga is something you can master and become proficient at doing simply by doing it every day and giving it some time.

Some Basic Yoga Poses and a sample sequence

Basic poses are ones that should be part of every yoga practice, and are poses you see being done in a typical yoga class. Let's start with warrior II. The three poses that follow can be strung together with Warrior II to make a good, short sequence.

Warrior II

- Stand and face the side of the mat. Spread feet approximately one meter apart.

- Point toes of right foot forward. Turn toes of left foot inward at an angle-be sure not to twist your knee.

- Bend right leg and bring knee is over ankle. Turn torso forward, in direction of right foot. Avoid tipping torso forward or sideways.

- Relax your shoulders, bring arms high overhead, hands shoulder-width apart; keep your neck and shoulders relaxed.

- *Repeat on other side.*

- Work to holding pose for 20 seconds. Thighs & buttocks create a Pelvic floor of support that holds weight of your torso. The thigh muscles are extended and engaged in this pose. Consult your physician before doing this pose. You'll likely be advised to keep hands at top of head and keep your stance less intense.

Revolved Triangle Pose

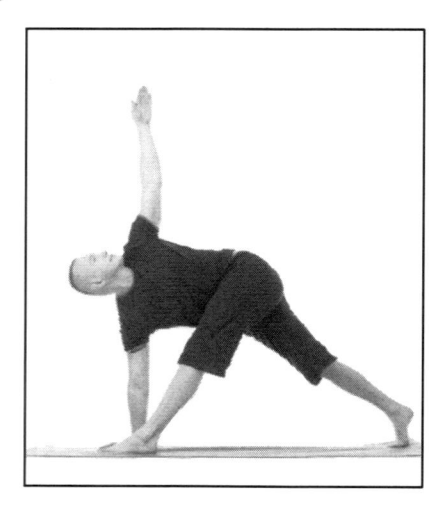

- Stand and face the side of the mat. Spread feet approximately one meter apart.

- Point toes of right foot forward. Turn toes of left foot inward at an angle-be sure not to twist your knee.

- Keep spine at full length and keep stomach muscles engaged as you fully extend your arms out, as if you were leaning gently against a wall behind you (you can use a wall in this manner to practice the pose and establish good alignment). Keeping your arms extended, tilt your torso rightward and down toward the floor.

- Bring your left hand downward so it can anchor softly on mat to the inside of your foot, or on top of your foot, or gripping your ankle. You can also anchor on a yoga block. Your right hand will be extended high in the air above your right shoulder, which gravitates backward as if you were leaning your whole torso against a wall (which you can do!)

- Work to holding pose 20 seconds.

- If you have high blood pressure, don't look upward-look ahead or down since your heart is above your head.

- *Repeat on other side.*

- This pose stretches the body from toe to neck, with intense work from upper leg to rib cage.

Half Moon Pose (Ardha Candrasana)

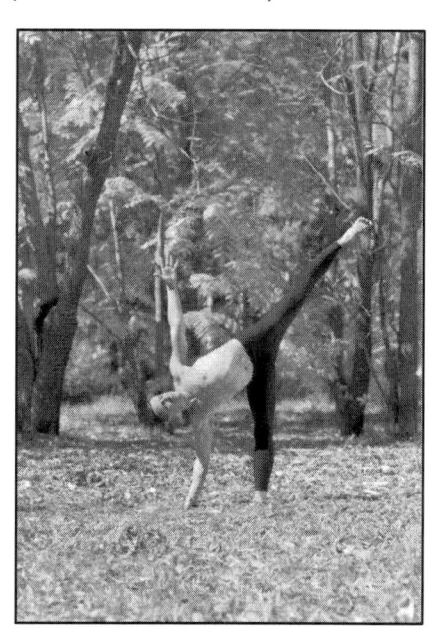

- There are at least several versions of a pose known as the Half Moon (Ardha Candrasana). This version was popularized by

Kirpalu yoga teacher Olivia Miller, authoress of the Yoga Deck. There is also a unique version of Half Moon that comes from the Iyengar discipline of Yoga.

- Stand with feet hip width apart.

- Move slowly into pose, letting torso be relaxed to allow easy breathing.

- Press your right foot down while letting your pelvis drift rightward as you lengthen the left side. Put your palms together overhead. Don't force your right side into folding-let it fold gradually as if you were pushing gently down to the floor or on a stack of pillows.

- Your left knee can bend slightly to enhance your balance and maintain a good level of comfort in the pose.

- Try to breathe slowly and keep your inhales and exhales the same length of time.

- *Repeat on other side.*

- This pose will reduce tightness in the sides and can help reduce lateral pelvic tilt.

Tree Pose (Vrksasana)

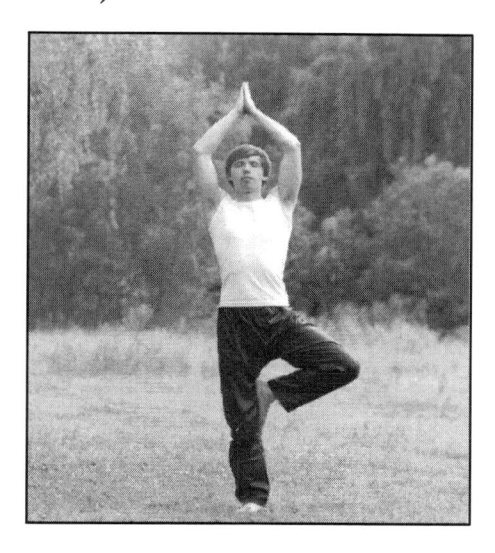

- This is a fun pose that will challenge you. It does a lot to even out the length of your muscles from your ankles up to your shoulders and will help you improve your balance over all. It is an excellent confidence builder that will also help you clear your head.

- Stand on your mat with your feet together. Shift your weight to your right foot. Bend your left leg and lift your left heel up off your mat. Here is where you make sure your abs aren't being lazy; you want your abs gently and fully engaged so they support your rib cage and keep you standing tall.

- Slowly turn you left knee outward so your heel touches inside of your right ankle, and then slowly take left foot/toes up off the mat by sliding the sole of the foot up the inside of your right leg.

- Don't push foot into knee joint.

- Left foot pushes firmly against interior of right leg, and in turn, right leg pushes equally back against left foot and creates equilibrium of balance. Keep your abs pulled in and keep standing tall to keep gravity working for you!

- Once balanced, slowly raise your arms overhead with palms facing each other until they touch. If you are struggling to balance, bring your hands touching together in front of chest.

- Hold position.

- *Repeat on other side.*

- This pose can help narrow one's center of gravity & can help even out length of muscles.

How to sequence more yoga poses

As you get into your own yoga practice, you'll be driven to practice more because it is going to make you feel good. Most new students quickly gain interest in expanding their practice because they quickly discover that they enjoy the poses and because yoga presents them with a different kind of challenge that motivates them.

You will soon find yourself looking for more poses to do and then you'll start creating your own daily routines. There are a few key things to remember when creating your own yoga sequences. Don't let the details drive you crazy, just remember these important things:

- **Make sure that transitioning from one pose to another is smooth.** You want your sequence to flow in a way that is not awkward for your mind or your body. You'll find many routines where a warrior and triangle pose are paired together in a sequence. Triangles and warriors are also sequenced with traditional lunge poses (see Sun Salutation sequence for information on lunges)

- **Make sure that poses which stretch one way are countered with poses that restore the length of stretched muscles.**

There are lots of examples of this kind of pose syncing. For example: triangle will stretch your hamstrings and lengthen your quads to plant your feet. Stretching these muscles is good, but it also can make the knee joints loose. In order to prevent this new-found looseness from letting the knees twist, we need to tweak the muscles around the knee joints to make sure the knees are still supported after we've made the hamstrings and quads longer. Warrior is the perfect countering pose because it flexes the quads, gluteus muscles and hamstrings to tighten them back up a bit and prevent the knee joints from getting too loose.

Sun Salutation-the most classic sequence you'll never stop doing

The best-known sequence of yoga poses is the Sun Salutation, also known as *Surya Namaskar* in the Sanskrit language. While this series of poses is believed to have once been an expression of worship in ancient times, it survives today because it works. It works incredibly well.

If you don't have time for a long yoga sequence, then do at least five Sun Salutations-this will make a huge difference in your day. Yoga poses not only work your muscles, they also work your emotional energy centers (known in yoga as *chakras*). The Sun Salutation series does an exceptional job at balancing your emotional energy centers as well as giving a comprehensive wake-up workout for your whole body.

For the Sun Salutation series, you'll get situated into each pose and then hold your full expression of the pose for at least 20 seconds. Get to know your muscles in each pose, and as you become more proficient, you can work to holding them longer. Proficiency also permits you to move quickly through the poses in the series as you hold them for shorter periods.

The beauty of the Sun Salutation is that you can go slow and hold each pose longer or go faster and move quickly through them in order to develop speed of focus.

Start with **Mountain Pose (Tadasana)**

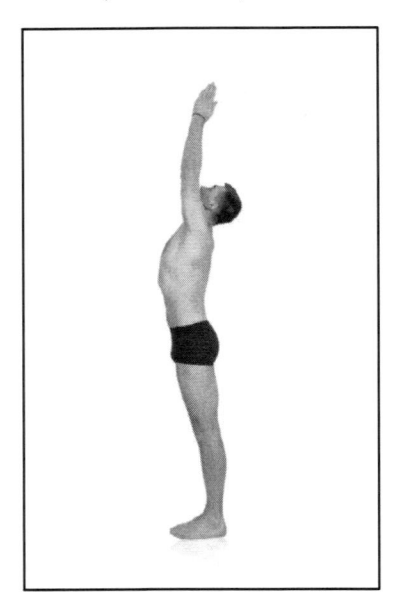

- Plant your feet, hip-width apart on your mat. Tighten your leg muscles around your leg bones gradually, starting from your ankles and moving up through your thighs.

- As your legs tighten, gently pull your abs inward and use your abs to lift your rib cage upward. Gently engage your lower back to lift your ribcage from behind.

- Take your hands overhead with your palms together. Keep lifting your hands upward, over the crown of your head. Let your shoulders be loose so they can follow your hands upward.

- Release yourself from the extended stretch before dropping hands to move into Standing Forward Bend.

Standing Forward Bend (Uttanasana)

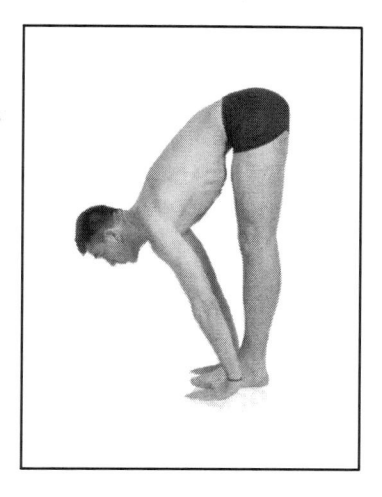

- Keep your knees unlocked and slightly bent as you flow into your forward bend. Catch elbows in your hands and begin bending from the upper back to the lower back.

- When into the forward bend, let your head be heavy, like a weight on a rope, and allow gravity to pull naturally on your head and your folded arms.

- Drop hands to mat and walk them forward to move into Downward Dog

*Take precautions if you have high blood pressure. Consult physician and don't bend over for more than ten second if you have high blood pressure unless approved by a physician.

Downward Dog (Adho Mukva Svanasana)

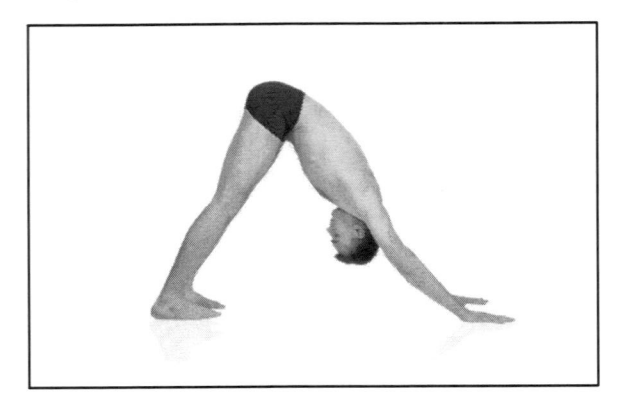

- Move into Downward Dog from Standing Forward Bend. Your hands should be shoulder-width apart and feet hip-width apart. Walk the hands forward. The legs and torso form a right angle.

- Hands should be anchored on mat with fingers spread wide. Pull your weight away from your anchored hands and send your weight to your hips. Your heels should gravitate toward the floor even if they aren't touching it.

- Let the back of your legs stretch intensely but don't lock your knees.

Forward lunge (not shown)

- From downward dog, lighten the weight on your right foot and then lunge your right foot forward. This will take some practice. You make your foot light in order to step forward into the lunge.

- You may need to adjust the position of your right foot once you lunge it forward. Your right ankle should be directly under your right knee so that shin is perpendicular to the floor. This prevents strain on the knee.

Plank Pose

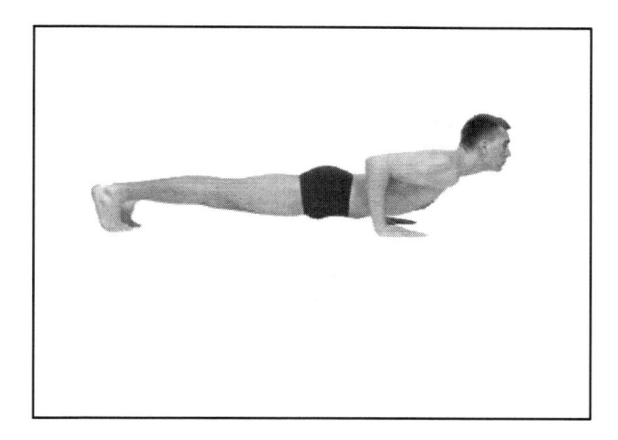

- Step your foot back from your lunge pose so you are in push-up position with your feet hip-width apart. Don't let your chest cave in between your shoulders too much as this puts strain on your rotator cuffs.

- The position is similar to the start of a press up whilst holding your weight off the ground.

- In plank position, push your hands down into the mat. This helps distribute your weight and enhances your ability to pull your core tight. Visualize your naval pulling inward toward your spine; it will help engage all four abdominal muscle groups.

- Come high up out of the balls of your feet and point your heels backward to keep your legs extended and engaged to help bear the weight.

This pose is a classic-it is often the subject of contests-folks like to see how long they can hold it. Long-held planks can result in over-fatiguing of the abs that support the back, so if you decide to do long planks (more than 30 seconds), proceed with caution.

Cobra Pose (Bhujangasana)

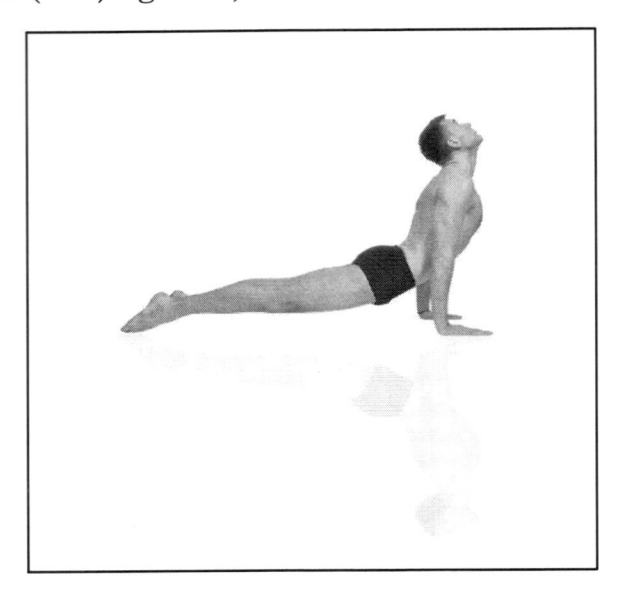

- From plan pose, uncurl your toes so that the tops of your feet are planted in the mat, then gently set knees down into mat. Using your abs, you will consciously and carefully lower your torso to the mat.

- Then make your pelvis light and lift your rib cage with your stomach. You will stretch your stomach muscles while they work and scoop your chest up between your shoulders as you inhale, letting your back bent very gently.

- Make sure your back isn't compressed as it bends in the Cobra Pose.

Child Pose (not shown)

- Relax out of Cobra Pose and pull your abs inward and come up on all fours. Then sit back onto your heels, with the tops of your feet in contact with the mat, and fold your stomach down onto your thighs. Extend your arms forward.

- The pose should be comfortable. If you need to make space between your knees for the pose to be comfortable, feel free to do it. You may also find you prefer to have your hands swept backwards.

- Rest your head on the mat and take full breaths. Let your spine relax and bend naturally.

Repeat the series, starting with Mountain Pose. But this time, you'll lunge the left foot forward for forward lunge. The rest of the series is the same as before.

The Sun Salutation is an example of a *Vinyasa*, which is just a fancy yoga word for *flow*. You'll find that the poses in Sun Salutation flow together very naturally and very easily. You can do multiple Sun Salutations to build cardio endurance.

Full Sequence - Sun Salutation

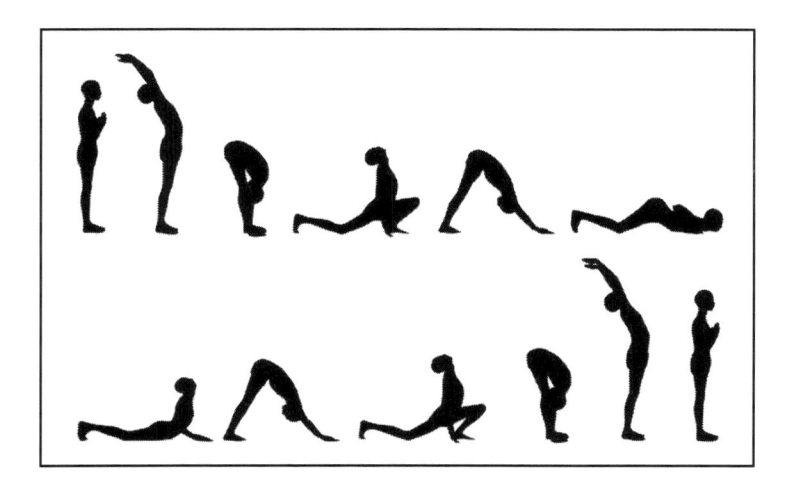

You can also do slow sun salutations to accentuate the aspects of each pose while still having a sequence of poses that that flows. Sun Salutations can also be adapted to include additional poses.

For example, you can easily move into a triangle or warrior pose from knee lunge. There are countless options, and you can create sequences that work for you. It will be pretty easy to get know how poses flow together just by trying what you feel like trying.

DEEP RELAXATION AND RECOVERY

You'll find that Sun Salutations and individual yoga poses make it much easier to relax. The yoga poses are the "magic switch", the one that you could never find when people told you again and again that you should "just relax".

As the muscles stretch out, a lot of positive things happen. Muscles cells function best when they are long. If they get compressed, they have a tougher time absorbing nutrients from the blood and getting rid of waste that needs to be expelled. Stretching in your yoga poses helps both these things happen.

As the muscles get stretched they are able to return to their normal length, and the cells that comprise the muscle tissue literally relax themselves. When tissues relax, they cease to secrete chemicals that they create when they are under stress or strain. Therefore, the brain no longer receives such chemicals as it would through your normal blood flow.

The brain begins to send its own, positive signals that tell the body to relax further. It produces "relaxation" chemicals that in turn relax the body tissue and muscles even further, and you move into a state of deep relaxation. In this state of deep relaxation, your body begins to heal and repair what needs to be fixed, and you enter a state of rebirth and recovery.

The Emotional Aspect of Yoga

Yoga does have a reputation for encouraging emotional expression. We need to clear things up here for the guys who are turned off by this idea. Yoga does not make you break down emotionally, nor does it make you become overly emotional or overly expressive. The effect of a good yoga session is quite the opposite-you gain confidence to express yourself and also gain the ability to turn off the tendency to be *too* expressive.

There really isn't anything complicated about the whole connection between yoga and self-expression. We don't want to get bogged down in the details of how it works, and we certainly don't want our yoga class to become a psychology lesson or a couch trip with a shrink. Let's look at it from a simple perspective, the way we'd look at a football play or the way we'd figure out how we're going to park a big truck in a small space.

When you start to contort yourself into a pose, such as revolved triangle or a sitting forward bend, you start to squish body parts together. It becomes harder to breath. You have to think about what you're doing. Even in a simpler pose like downward dog, you're going to be challenged. Speaking of downward dog, just ask any athlete who doesn't do much stretching, or better yet, just ask yourself!

If you're not used to stretching your hamstrings, then your hamstrings are going to be very tight. When it comes to hamstrings, as it does with any other muscle, tightness translates to shortness of the muscle. So, even a simple pose like downward dog will be a big challenge for a person new to yoga. Pardon the pun, but in short, there's a lot of work to be done while you are standing still in your downward dog.

It's about being honest with yourself

When you get into a pose and find that your muscles are really tight, there's no room for bull. You have to be totally honest with yourself. If you can't go further into the pose, you face that fact head-on. You have to take yourself to the edge of your happy place, your comfort zone. You can't lie to yourself about it. Once you go past the point where the pose is easy, you feel the tug on your muscles.

What are the perks to feeling the tightness and thinking it might be a bit like torture? For starters, you can't help but develop a deeper connection with that muscle and that muscle group. You start to get to know your body on a much higher level. In getting to know your body, you get to know yourself. The idea is very simple. As you start to stretch your hamstrings, you start to realize what hurts when your hamstrings are tight; you get connected to the rest of your body.

Tight hamstrings, of course, will pull your pelvis down from behind and over extend your back muscles. You start to reflect on how you feel after a pose, and suddenly, you're more connected with yourself as you've learned how your different muscles are connected. This means you start to stamp out the unknowns that kept you guessing. Fear of the unknown is the most common type of fear we will experience throughout life; it's human nature to fear what we can't understand.

As we eliminate the unknowns of our body, we eliminate the unknowns within ourselves. That translates to a big increase in self-confidence. So, as you can see, we've had a yogi revelation of sorts, right here and now, and it will be even better when you try downward dog for yourself. Yoga just happens to do a great job getting you in touch with the basics. You stretch out tight muscles; you get a better connection to your body. Once you have a better connection to your body, you get a better connection to yourself. A better connection means stamping out some unknowns, and that will develop your self-confidence. Greater confidence leads to more strength and more resolve.

All of this helps you get to a calmer state of mind and a calmer state of being. You become more comfortable with yourself, and so you can't help but be more comfortable expressing yourself and expressing your true feelings in your actions. That's all anyone is really talking about when they talk about the emotional freedom that yoga gives them.

It will be your gift as you get onto your yoga mat. It will not make you weak; it will not make you unstable; you won't turn into a crazy person. Quite the opposite, you'll feel better than you've felt in a long time and you'll be motivated to practice yoga more often. You might go through a short period of obsession with your yoga practice because you've never felt the way you do before you started doing yoga.

Your initial obsession is part of the process. As your practice grows and as you master some specific poses, you'll start to channel this energy into your workout and you'll start to take this energy beyond your yoga mat. The initial obsession can't be helped with most students; it just has to run its course.

Why does this happen? Again, the answer is quite simple. Yoga reconnects you to the basic emotions that you felt when you were a kid. Remember when you didn't worry about doing stuff you wanted to do because it sounded fun? Remember liking yourself for who you were and not questioning it and not analyzing who you were before deciding you liked who you were? All those feelings return to you when you get going with your yoga.

There's no need to overthink your yoga practice. Follow the simple instructions for the poses so you can practice safely. The rest will come to you.

SUMMARY

It won't take you long to seek more information on more yoga poses. Practice on your own to become familiar with the basics. If you venture out to a class, remind yourself that people won't be hanging out staring at you-they won't have time. Just like you, they will have to pay attention to the instructor and to their own poses.

Yoga for men is still a new thing in the fitness world. Any decent gym or yoga studio will be open to hearing your feedback-and suggestions-of having yoga classes for men.

Your yoga practice will compliment your gym workouts and help you with many of the traditional sports we know and live, like skiing, golf and running, just to name a few.

Yoga has transformed my body, mind and life. I hope that you're able to reap the same rewards.

Best wishes

Jake

YOGA RESOURCES FOR BEGINNERS

Daily Cup of Yoga
www.dailycupofyoga.com

Yoga Paws
www.yogapaws.com

Yoga Dork
www.yogadork.com

Yoga Mint
www.yogamint.com

USA Today 09-26-03
http://usatoday30.usatoday.com/news/health/spotlighthealth/2003-09-26-jabbar_x.htm

Postgame.com December, 2013
http://www.thepostgame.com/blog/eye-performance/201312/kareem-abdul-jabbar-yoga-lakers-nba-basketball-pioneer

Stack.com 12-09-12
http://www.stack.com/2012/09/17/yoga-athletes/

ABC News Oct 14, 2014
http://abcnews.go.com/Business/story?id=86918

Media Bistro.com
http://www.mediabistro.com/QA-John-Capouya-a808.html

Printed in Great Britain
by Amazon.co.uk, Ltd.,
Marston Gate.